TETRACYCLINE HYDROCLORIDE MANUAL

Nathan Bosso

Copyright © 2024 by Nathan Bosso. All rights reserved.

Disclaimer

The data gave on this stage is to instructive and educational purposes as it were. It isn't expected as a substitute for proficient clinical counsel, conclusion, or treatment. Continuously look for the counsel of your doctor or other qualified wellbeing supplier with any inquiries you might have in regards to an ailment. Never ignore proficient clinical guidance or postpone in looking for it in light of something you have perused on this stage.

Table of Contents

CHAPTER ONE;......................5

Introduction to tetracycline.........5

CHAPTER TWO.........................12

Uses of tetracycline................12

CHAPTER THREE.................17

Side Effects tetracycline........17

Chapter FOUR.........................21

Dosage Guidelines for tetracycline 21

CHAPTER FIVE.......................26

Interaction on Tetracyclines...26

CHAPTER SIX..........................31

FAQ..31

CHAPTER ONEs

Introduction to tetracycline

What Are Tetracycline's?

tetracycline are a class of broad-spectrum antibiotics known for their ability to inhibit bacterial protein synthesis. They are derived from the Streptomyces genus of bacteria and are effective against a wide range of gram-positive and gram-negative bacteria, as well as some protozoa. Their unique mechanism of action makes them a valuable tool in the treatment of various infectious diseases.

Historical Background

The discovery of tetracycline's dates back to the late 1940s, when they were isolated from the fermentation products of *Streptomyces aureofaciens*. The first antibiotic in this class, tetracycline, was introduced in 1948. Over the years, several derivatives have been developed, including doxycycline, minocycline, and tigecycline, each with specific pharmacological properties and clinical applications.

Initially, tetracycline were heralded as wonder drugs, effectively treating diseases such as pneumonia, urinary tract infections, and acne. Their ability to penetrate tissues and remain effective in various body fluids further enhanced their appeal in clinical practice.

Importance in Medicine

tetracycline play a crucial role in modern medicine for several reasons:

Broad Spectrum of Activity: They are effective against a diverse range of pathogens, including those resistant to other antibiotics, making them valuable in treating infections where other options may be limited.

Versatility: tetracycline are used to treat a variety of conditions, from bacterial infections and acne to certain parasitic diseases like malaria. This versatility extends their relevance across multiple medical specialties.

Impact on Public Health: tetracycline have been instrumental in managing public health concerns, including outbreaks of diseases like Lyme disease and rickettsia infections.

Veterinary Applications: Beyond human medicine, tetracycline are widely used in veterinary medicine to treat infections in livestock and pets, contributing to animal health and food safety.

Research and Development: Ongoing research continues to explore new uses and formulations of tetracycline, including their potential anti-inflammatory properties and applications in chronic diseases.

Despite the emergence of antibiotic resistance, tetracycline remain a cornerstone of treatment protocols in various settings. Understanding their history, mechanisms, and current applications provides essential context for their continued use in medicine today.

The introduction of tetracycline marked a significant advancement in the fight against infectious diseases. As we explore their chemical structure, mechanisms of action, clinical uses, and challenges in the following chapters, it becomes evident that these antibiotics remain a vital component of contemporary healthcare. Their versatility and broad-spectrum efficacy underscore the need for ongoing education and research in optimizing their use in both human and veterinary medicine.

CHAPTER TWO

Chemical Structure and Mechanism of Action

Chemical Composition

tetracycline are a group of antibiotics characterized by a four-ring polycyclic structure. This chemical backbone is essential for their biological activity and is responsible for their ability to bind to ribosomes and inhibit protein synthesis. The core structure can be modified with various side chains, leading to different derivatives, each with unique pharmacokinetic properties.

Key Features of the Tetracycline Structure:

- **Four Hydrocarbon Rings**: The central structure consists of four fused rings, designated A, B, C, and D. This arrangement is critical for their interaction with bacterial ribosomes.
- **Functional Groups**: Various functional groups attached to the rings, such as hydroxyl (-OH) and dimethyl amino groups, contribute to the solubility and effectiveness of each tetracycline derivative.
- **Chirality**: Many tetracycline possess multiple stereo centers, which can affect their pharmacological properties and biological activity.

How tetracycline Work

Mechanism of Action

The primary mechanism of action for tetracycline involves the inhibition of bacterial protein synthesis. They achieve this by binding to the 30S ribosomal subunit, a crucial component of the bacterial ribosome. This interaction disrupts the translation process, preventing the synthesis of essential proteins necessary for bacterial growth and reproduction.

Steps in the Mechanism:

Binding to Ribosomes: tetracycline enter bacterial cells through passive diffusion and active transport. Once inside, they bind to the 30S ribosomal subunit.

Inhibition of tRNA Binding: By binding to the ribosome, tetracycline block the attachment of aminoacyl-tRNA to the mRNA-ribosome complex. This step is vital for translating genetic information into proteins.

Disruption of Protein Synthesis: The inhibition of tRNA binding ultimately leads to the cessation of protein synthesis, which is essential for bacterial growth and reproduction.

Spectrum of Activity

tetracycline exhibit broad-spectrum activity, affecting a variety of both gram-positive and gram-negative bacteria, as well as atypical pathogens. This makes them effective against:

- **Common Bacterial Infections**: Streptococcus pneumonia, Staphylococcus aureus (including some MRSA strains), and Escherichia coli.
- **Atypical Pathogens**: Mycoplasma pneumonia, Chlamydia species, and Rickettsia species.
- **Protozoa**: Some tetracycline are also effective against certain protozoal infections, such as those caused by *Plasmodium* (malaria).

Resistance Mechanisms

While tetracycline are powerful antibiotics, resistance has emerged as a significant challenge. Bacteria can develop resistance through various mechanisms, including:

- **Efflux Pumps**: Some bacteria can expel tetracycline from their cells before they can exert their effects.
- **Ribosomal Protection**: Certain proteins produced by resistant bacteria can bind to the ribosome and protect it from tetracycline binding.

- **Enzymatic Modification**: Bacteria may produce enzymes that chemically modify tetracycline, rendering them ineffective.

The unique chemical structure of tetracycline underpins their potent antibiotic action, primarily through the inhibition of bacterial protein synthesis. Understanding this mechanism is crucial for healthcare professionals to effectively utilize these antibiotics and address the challenges posed by antibiotic resistance. In the next chapters, we will explore the various types of tetracycline, their clinical uses, and the implications of their resistance patterns.

CHAPTER TWO

Uses of tetracycline

tetracycline are versatile antibiotics with a broad spectrum of activity, making them suitable for treating various infections across multiple medical specialties. This chapter explores the key clinical applications of tetracycline, highlighting their efficacy, common indications, and unique properties.

Bacterial Infections

Respiratory Tract Infections

- **Conditions**: tetracycline, particularly doxycycline and minocycline, are effective against common pathogens causing community-acquired pneumonia, such as *Streptococcus pneumonias* and *Mycoplasma pneumonias*.
- **Usage**: Often prescribed as a first-line treatment or in cases of penicillin allergy.

Skin and Soft Tissue Infections

- **Conditions**: tetracycline are effective against skin infections caused by *Staphylococcus aureus* and *Propionibacterium acnes*.

- **Usage**: Minocycline and doxycycline are commonly used to treat acne and other inflammatory skin conditions.

Acne Treatment

Mechanism

- tetracycline, especially doxycycline and minocycline, reduce inflammation and inhibit bacterial growth, addressing both the inflammatory and non-inflammatory aspects of acne.

Usage

- Often used in combination with topical treatments for moderate to severe acne. Long-term use may be required to achieve optimal results.

Lyme Disease and Other Tick-Borne Illnesses

Lyme Disease

- **Pathogen**: *Borrelia burgdorferi*.
- **Usage**: Doxycycline is the preferred treatment for early Lyme disease due to its efficacy and ability to penetrate tissues.

Other Tick-Borne Diseases

- tetracycline are also effective against conditions like anaplasmosis and ehrlichiosis, making them valuable in regions where these diseases are endemic.

Rickettsia Infections

Overview

- tetracycline are the treatment of choice for rickettsia infections, such as Rocky Mountain spotted fever and typhus.

Usage

- Early initiation of doxycycline is critical for effective treatment and to reduce morbidity and mortality.

Malaria Prevention and Treatment

Overview

- Doxycycline is used as a prophylactic agent against malaria in travelers to endemic regions.

Usage

- Administered before, during, and after travel to high-risk areas to prevent infection, particularly in combination with other antimalarial drugs.

Chlamydia Infections

Overview

- tetracycline, particularly doxycycline, are effective against *Chlamydia trachomatis*.

Usage

- Doxycycline is often prescribed as a first-line treatment for uncomplicated chlamydial infections, typically administered over a seven-day course.

Periodontal Disease

Overview

- Doxycycline can be used in the management of chronic periodontitis.

Usage

- As an adjunct to scaling and root planning, doxycycline may reduce pocket depth and promote periodontal healing.

Other Clinical Applications

Anthrax

- Doxycycline is effective against *Bacillus anthracic*, making it a crucial part of treatment and post-exposure prophylaxis.

Plague

- tetracycline can be used in the treatment of infections caused by *Yersinia pestis*.

Intra-abdominal Infections

- Tigecycline is indicated for complicated intra-abdominal infections, especially those caused by resistant organisms.

tetracycline are indispensable in the treatment of various bacterial infections, from common respiratory illnesses to complex conditions like Lyme disease and rickettsia infections. Their unique properties, including anti-inflammatory effects and broad-spectrum activity, make them a valuable tool in modern medicine. As we move forward, the next chapters will cover pharmacokinetics, side effects, and the growing concern of antibiotic resistance related to tetracycline.

CHAPTER THREE

Side Effects tetracycline

While tetracycline are effective antibiotics, they are associated with a range of side effects and contraindications that healthcare providers must consider when prescribing these medications. This chapter outlines the common and serious side effects, contraindications, and important drug interactions associated with tetracycline.

Common Side Effects

Gastrointestinal Disturbances

- **Symptoms**: Nausea, vomiting, diarrhea, and abdominal discomfort are common.
- **Mechanism**: These effects are often due to irritation of the gastrointestinal tract and alterations in gut flora.

Photosensitivity

- **Symptoms**: Increased sensitivity to sunlight can lead to sunburn or skin rashes.
- **Advice**: Patients are advised to use sunscreen and protective clothing while taking tetracycline.

Allergic Reactions

- **Symptoms**: Rashes, urticaria, and in rare cases, anaphylaxis.
- **Management**: Immediate discontinuation of the drug and treatment of the allergic reaction are essential.

Discoloration of Teeth

- **Symptoms**: tetracycline can cause permanent yellow or gray discoloration of teeth in children and pregnant women.
- **Advice**: Use is contraindicated during pregnancy and in children under the age of 8.

Serious Adverse Effects

Hepatotoxicity

- **Symptoms**: Elevated liver enzymes, jaundice, and liver dysfunction.
- **Management**: Regular monitoring of liver function tests is recommended, particularly in patients with pre-existing liver conditions.

Intracranial Hypertension

- **Symptoms**: Headache, visual disturbances, and symptoms similar to increased intracranial pressure.
- **Advice**: Discontinue the medication if symptoms occur, especially in patients with a history of intracranial hypertension.

Superinfection

- **Symptoms**: New infections caused by resistant organisms, such as Clostridium difficile-associated diarrhea.
- **Management**: Monitor for signs of Superinfection, and treat accordingly if it occurs.

Contraindications

Pregnancy and Lactation

- **Reason**: tetracycline can affect fetal development, particularly in tooth and bone formation.
- **Advice**: Alternative antibiotics should be considered for pregnant or breastfeeding women.

Pediatric Patients

- **Reason**: The use of tetracycline is contraindicated in children under 8 years due to the risk of dental discoloration and potential effects on bone growth.

- **Advice**: Alternatives should be explored for treating infections in this age group.

Hypersensitivity

- **Reason**: Patients with a known allergy to tetracycline should avoid these medications.
- **Advice**: Review patient history for any allergic reactions to antibiotics.

Drug Interactions

Antacids and Divalent/Trivalent Cations

- **Impact**: Calcium, magnesium, and iron can bind to tetracycline, reducing their absorption and effectiveness.
- **Advice**: Patients should be advised to space the administration of these supplements or medications by at least 2-3 hours from tetracycline doses.

Oral Contraceptives

- **Impact**: tetracycline may reduce the effectiveness of oral contraceptives, leading to potential contraceptive failure.
- **Advice**: Patients should be counseled on additional contraceptive measures during treatment.

Warfarin and Other Anticoagulants

- **Impact**: tetracycline may enhance the anticoagulant effects of warfarin, increasing the risk of bleeding.
- **Advice**: Regular monitoring of INR levels is recommended for patients on warfarin during tetracycline therapy.

Awareness of the potential side effects and contraindications of tetracycline is crucial for safe and effective prescribing. By carefully considering these factors, healthcare providers can minimize risks and optimize treatment outcomes. In the following chapters, we will examine resistance mechanisms and the future implications of tetracycline use in clinical practice.

CHAPTER FOUR

Dosage Guidelines for tetracycline

Proper administration and dosage of tetracycline are critical for maximizing their efficacy while minimizing the risk of side effects and resistance development. This chapter provides an overview of general administration guidelines, specific dosage recommendations for various tetracycline derivatives, and considerations for special populations.

General Administration Guidelines

Route of Administration

- **Oral**: Most tetracycline, including doxycycline, minocycline, and tetracycline, are available in oral forms (tablets and capsules).
- **Intravenous**: Doxycycline can also be administered intravenously in hospital settings for more severe infections.

Timing with Food and Other Medications

- **Empty Stomach**: Tetracycline should be taken on an empty stomach (1 hour before or 2 hours after meals) to optimize absorption. Doxycycline and

minocycline can be taken with food if gastrointestinal upset occurs but may have slightly reduced absorption.
- **Avoiding Antacids**: Patients should be advised to avoid antacids and supplements containing calcium, magnesium, or iron within 2-3 hours of taking tetracycline, as these can form insoluble complexes that inhibit absorption.

Duration of Therapy

- **Course Length**: The duration of treatment varies depending on the infection being treated, generally ranging from 7 to 14 days for most acute infections. Chronic conditions like acne may require longer-term therapy, sometimes for several months.

Dosage Recommendations by Tetracycline Derivative

Tetracycline

- **Adult Dosage**: 250-500 mg orally every 6 hours.
- **Pediatric Dosage**: 10-20 mg/kg/day in divided doses, not exceeding 1 g/day.
- **Special Considerations**: Dosage adjustments may be necessary for patients with renal impairment.

Doxycycline

- **Adult Dosage**:
    - **Initial Dose**: 100 mg orally or intravenously on the first day.
    - **Maintenance Dose**: 100 mg orally or intravenously every 12 hours.
- **Pediatric Dosage**: 2 mg/kg on the first day, then 1 mg/kg daily, not exceeding 100 mg/day.
- **Special Considerations**: Doxycycline is preferred in patients with renal impairment due to its alternative excretion route.

Minocycline

- **Adult Dosage**:
    - **Initial Dose**: 200 mg orally or intravenously on the first day.
    - **Maintenance Dose**: 100 mg orally or intravenously every 12 hours.
- **Pediatric Dosage**: 4 mg/kg on the first day, followed by 2 mg/kg daily, not exceeding 200 mg/day.
- **Special Considerations**: Caution in patients with hepatic impairment is advised.

Tigecycline

- **Adult Dosage**:
    - **Initial Dose**: 100 mg intravenously.

- o **Maintenance Dose**: 50 mg intravenously every 12 hours.
- **Special Considerations**: Not recommended for use in bloodstream infections due to low serum concentrations.

Special Populations

Pregnant Women

- **Contraindication**: tetracycline should generally be avoided during pregnancy due to risks of fetal harm, including tooth discoloration and skeletal abnormalities.

Pediatric Patients

- **Contraindication**: tetracycline are contraindicated in children under 8 years due to potential effects on dental and bone development.

Elderly Patients

- **Considerations**: Caution is advised in prescribing tetracycline to elderly patients, especially those with renal or hepatic impairment, as they may be more susceptible to adverse effects.

Monitoring and Follow-Up

Laboratory Monitoring

- **Liver Function Tests**: Regular monitoring of liver function may be necessary in patients on prolonged tetracycline therapy.
- **Renal Function**: Assess renal function periodically, especially in patients receiving long-term treatment or those with existing renal impairment.

Clinical Monitoring

- **Efficacy**: Regular follow-up appointments to assess treatment response and side effects are essential. If there is no clinical improvement within a few days, consider reevaluation for alternative therapies or resistance.

Adhering to proper administration and dosage guidelines for tetracycline is essential for effective treatment outcomes. By considering individual patient factors and the specific characteristics of each tetracycline derivative, healthcare providers can optimize therapy while minimizing the risk of side effects and resistance. In the next chapter, we will explore future directions in tetracycline research and the ongoing evolution of their use in clinical practice.

CHAPTER FIVE

Interaction on Tetracyclines

Tetracyclines, known for their broad-spectrum antibiotic properties, are widely used to treat various bacterial infections. However, understanding the long-term interactions and implications of tetracycline therapy is essential for optimizing patient outcomes. This chapter discusses the long-term use of tetracyclines, potential interactions with other medications and conditions, and considerations for patient management.

Long-Term Use of Tetracyclines

Indications for Long-Term Therapy

Tetracyclines may be prescribed for extended durations in several conditions, including:

- **Chronic Acne**: Often treated with doxycycline or minocycline to reduce inflammation and bacterial load.
- **Rosacea**: Low-dose doxycycline is used to manage inflammatory lesions.
- **Periodontal Disease**: Long-term doxycycline can aid in managing chronic periodontitis.

- **Prophylaxis**: Doxycycline is used for malaria prophylaxis in travelers and as a preventive measure against certain infections in at-risk populations.

Monitoring During Long-Term Therapy

- **Adverse Effects**: Patients on long-term tetracycline therapy should be monitored for gastrointestinal disturbances, hepatotoxicity, and skin reactions.
- **Resistance Development**: Regular assessment for signs of treatment failure or infection recurrence can indicate potential resistance.

Drug Interactions with Tetracyclines

Common Drug Interactions

Tetracyclines interact with several classes of medications, impacting their effectiveness and safety:

- **Antacids and Supplements**: Divalent and trivalent cations (calcium, magnesium, iron) can form complexes with tetracyclines, reducing their absorption. Patients should be advised to take these substances at least 2-3 hours apart.

- **Oral Contraceptives**: Tetracyclines may reduce the effectiveness of oral contraceptives, leading to potential contraceptive failure. Women should be counseled on alternative contraceptive methods while on tetracyclines.
- **Anticoagulants**: Tetracyclines can enhance the effects of anticoagulants like warfarin, increasing the risk of bleeding. Regular monitoring of INR levels is advised for patients taking both medications.

Impact of Comorbid Conditions

Certain chronic conditions can also interact with tetracycline therapy:

- **Renal Impairment**: Tetracyclines, particularly those eliminated by the kidneys, may require dose adjustments in patients with renal insufficiency to avoid accumulation and toxicity.
- **Hepatic Impairment**: Caution is needed with tetracyclines in patients with liver disease, as they may have altered metabolism and excretion.

Long-Term Implications of Tetracycline Use

Development of Antibiotic Resistance

- **Mechanisms of Resistance**: Prolonged use of tetracyclines can lead to the emergence of resistant

bacterial strains through mechanisms such as efflux pumps and ribosomal protection.
- **Impact on Treatment Options**: Increased resistance may limit the effectiveness of tetracyclines and other classes of antibiotics, complicating treatment for common infections.

Effects on Microbiome

- **Microbiota Disruption**: Long-term tetracycline therapy can disrupt the normal gut microbiota, leading to issues such as Clostridium difficile infection (CDI) and other gastrointestinal disturbances.
- **Restoration of Microbiome**: Patients on prolonged tetracycline therapy may benefit from probiotics or dietary modifications to support gut health.

Lifestyle and Dietary Modifications

- **Dietary Adjustments**: Patients should be advised on how to take tetracyclines correctly, including the timing of food and supplements to maximize absorption.
- **Sun Protection**: Due to the risk of photosensitivity, patients should be advised to use sunscreen and protective clothing when exposed to sunlight.

Long-term tetracycline therapy can be effective for managing chronic conditions, but it carries significant implications, including the risk of resistance, interactions with other medications, and potential side effects. By understanding these factors and implementing appropriate monitoring and patient education strategies, healthcare providers can enhance treatment outcomes and ensure the safe use of tetracyclines. In the next chapter, we will explore future directions in tetracycline research and their evolving role in clinical practice.

CHAPTER SIX

FAQ

Frequently Asked Questions (FAQ) about Tetracyclines

What are tetracyclines?

Tetracyclines are a class of broad-spectrum antibiotics that inhibit bacterial protein synthesis. They are effective against a variety of bacteria, making them useful for treating a range of infections, including respiratory infections, acne, and certain tick-borne diseases.

How do tetracyclines work?

Tetracyclines work by binding to the 30S ribosomal subunit of bacteria, preventing the attachment of aminoacyl-tRNA to the mRNA-ribosome complex. This inhibition stops protein synthesis, ultimately leading to bacterial growth inhibition.

What are the common types of tetracyclines?

The main tetracyclines include:

- **Tetracycline**: The original drug in the class.

- **Doxycycline**: Known for its high bioavailability and longer half-life.
- **Minocycline**: Noted for its anti-inflammatory properties.
- **Tigecycline**: A newer derivative used for multidrug-resistant infections.

What are the common side effects of tetracyclines?

Common side effects include:

- Gastrointestinal disturbances (nausea, vomiting, diarrhea)
- Photosensitivity (increased risk of sunburn)
- Allergic reactions (rashes, itching)
- Tooth discoloration in children and during pregnancy

Are there any contraindications for tetracyclines?

Yes, tetracyclines are generally contraindicated in:

- Pregnant women (risk of fetal harm)
- Children under 8 years (risk of tooth discoloration)
- Patients with known hypersensitivity to tetracyclines

How should tetracyclines be taken?

Tetracyclines are usually taken orally. They should be taken on an empty stomach (1 hour before or 2 hours after meals) for optimal absorption. Patients should also avoid taking them with antacids or supplements containing calcium, magnesium, or iron.

What should I do if I miss a dose of tetracycline?

If you miss a dose, take it as soon as you remember. If it's almost time for your next dose, skip the missed dose and resume your regular schedule. Do not take two doses at once.

Can I drink alcohol while taking tetracyclines?

While moderate alcohol consumption may not significantly affect tetracycline effectiveness, it's generally advisable to limit alcohol intake, especially since both alcohol and tetracyclines can irritate the stomach.

What should I do if I experience severe side effects?

If you experience severe side effects, such as difficulty breathing, severe rash, or signs of liver dysfunction (e.g., jaundice, dark urine), seek medical attention immediately and discontinue the medication.

How does antibiotic resistance affect tetracyclines?

Overuse or misuse of tetracyclines can lead to antibiotic resistance, making these medications less effective against certain bacterial strains. It's important to use tetracyclines judiciously and follow healthcare provider recommendations.

Can tetracyclines interact with other medications?

Yes, tetracyclines can interact with several medications, including:

- Antacids and supplements (calcium, magnesium, iron)
- Oral contraceptives (may reduce effectiveness)
- Anticoagulants (increased risk of bleeding)

Always inform your healthcare provider about all medications you are taking.

Is it safe to use tetracyclines long-term?

Long-term use of tetracyclines can be appropriate for certain conditions (e.g., chronic acne) but requires careful monitoring for side effects, resistance, and other interactions. Always discuss **long-term therapy with your healthcare provider.**

What are the signs of an allergic reaction to tetracyclines?

Signs of an allergic reaction may include hives, rash, itching, swelling (especially of the face, tongue, or throat), and difficulty breathing. If you experience any of these symptoms, seek immediate medical attention.

If you have any additional questions or concerns about tetracyclines, consult your healthcare provider for personalized advice and information.

www.ingramcontent.com/pod-product-compliance
Lightning Source LLC
Chambersburg PA
CBHW070956220526
45471CB00007B/3061